YOUR KNOWLEDGE HAS VALUE

AF140342

- We will publish your bachelor's and master's thesis, essays and papers

- Your own eBook and book - sold worldwide in all relevant shops

- Earn money with each sale

Upload your text at www.GRIN.com and publish for free

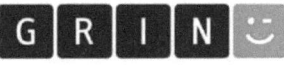

Bibliographic information published by the German National Library:

The German National Library lists this publication in the National Bibliography; detailed bibliographic data are available on the Internet at http://dnb.dnb.de .

Imprint:

Copyright © 2016 GRIN Verlag, Open Publishing GmbH
Print and binding: Books on Demand GmbH, Norderstedt Germany
ISBN: 9783668612105

This book at GRIN:

https://www.grin.com/document/384371

Patrick Kimuyu

Interventions Used To Reduce College Statistics Anxiety

Critical Review of Literature

GRIN Publishing

GRIN - Your knowledge has value

Since its foundation in 1998, GRIN has specialized in publishing academic texts by students, college teachers and other academics as e-book and printed book. The website www.grin.com is an ideal platform for presenting term papers, final papers, scientific essays, dissertations and specialist books.

Visit us on the internet:

http://www.grin.com/

http://www.facebook.com/grincom

http://www.twitter.com/grin_com

Critical Review of Literature on Interventions Used To Reduce College Statistics

Anxiety

Name: Patrick Kimuyu

Introduction...2

Defining Statistics Anxiety...3

Distinguishing Statistics Anxiety from Math Anxiety..3

Antecedents of Statistics Anxiety...5

The Need for Intervention...7

Interventions for Reducing Statistics Anxiety in College Students............................8

Use of Live Vicarious Experience Presentation...9

Value-Reappraisal...10

Use of Humor...11

Use of Instructor Immediacy...12

Religious Motivation...13

Use of Multifaceted Teaching Framework..14

In-Class Collaborative Problem Solving...14

Combined Instructional Strategies..16

Summary of Literature on Statistics Anxiety Interventions......................................16

References..18

Introduction

Statistics anxiety has become an issue of concern in higher education due to its implications on teaching and learning (Chiou, Wang & Lee, 2014; Macheski, Buhrmann, Lowney & Bush, 2008). In retrospect, the trends of statistics anxiety are quite alarming. This aspect is evidenced by Onwuegbuzie and Wilson (2003) who report that statistic anxiety affects 80% of behavioral and social sciences students. They also report that most degree programs require students to enroll in quantitative research and statistics courses as part of their training. These statistic courses are reported to evoke anxiety-provoking experiences among students (Onwuegbuzie & Wilson, 2003). Similarly, Macher et al. (2013) reaffirm that statistics courses have been found to be the major source of anxiety in student's curriculum. Further evidence is provided by Dykeman's (2011) study which investigated the levels of anxiety between students in statistic courses and those in other education courses. Results of this study revealed that statistics students had lower self-efficacy ($p<.01$) and higher levels of anxiety ($p< .05$) compared to other students. As such, research on statistics anxiety has focused on the causes, as well as the statistics anxiety-reducing interventions. In this context, it is worth noting that statistics anxiety, as a construct, is different from math anxiety, which has been discussed extensively by researchers. Factor analysis reveals that statistics anxiety comprises of six dimensions: fear of statistics teacher, interpretation anxiety, computational self-concept, worth of statistics, fear of asking for help, and test and class anxiety (Cruise, Cash & Bolton, 1985). In contrast, mathematics anxiety has one dimension: fear of mathematics (Hak, 2014). Therefore, this literature review aims at discussing the interventions that can reduce statistics anxiety among college students. To achieve this objective, a concise definition of statistics anxiety, as well as, the distinction between statistics anxiety and math anxiety is provided as the scientific rationale why the focus of this discussion is on interventions that reduce statistics anxiety, but not math anxiety in general.

Defining Statistics Anxiety

Over the decades, extensive research on the principal aspects anxiety in college students, especially in mathematics and statistics education has led to a consensus on the definition of these two phenomena (Cruise, Cash & Bolton, 1985; Fennema & Sherman, 1976). It is universally acceptable to define statistics anxiety as a form of anxiety resulting from encountering statistics at any time. In general, Cruise, Cash and Bolton (1985) summarize the definition of statistics anxiety as "the feelings of anxiety encountered when taking a statistics course or doing a statistical analysis; that is, gathering, processing, and interpret[ing]" (p. 92). As such, statistics definition appears to be different from that of mathematics anxiety. Fennema and Sherman (1976) defined mathematics anxiety as "the feelings of anxiety, dread, nervousness, and associated bodily symptoms related to doing mathematics" (p. 324).

Distinguishing Statistics Anxiety from Math Anxiety

From a critical perspective, statistics anxiety and mathematics anxiety are two distinct constructs. Overall, it is apparent that mathematics anxiety, as a construct, which results from the manipulation of numbers depends solely on mathematics reasoning. In contrast, statistics anxiety is characterized by an array of emotional reactions arising from any form of encounter to statistics (Onwuegbuzie, 2004). As such, it implies that statistics anxiety is more cognitive in nature, meaning that it requires more verbal reasoning than mathematics reasoning (Zerbolio, 1999). This aspect is acknowledged by Baloglu (2004) whose review of literature showed that there are significant differences between statistics and mathematics based on the cognitive process.

A clear distinction between statistics anxiety and mathematics anxiety is provided by one prospective study that was conducted recently by Malik (2014) to investigate whether these constructs are similar or different from one another. In principle, Malik (2014) sought to clear the old-age misconception among researchers, most of whom regard statistics anxiety as mathematics anxiety. As such, he wanted to substantiate that his point of view that these constructs are different; thus, they require to be dealt with in different perspectives.

In this study, the Malik (2014) used the highly validated instruments of Students' statistics anxiety scale (SSAS) and students' mathematics anxiety scale (SMAS) to investigate different variables which are associated with the levels of two constructs among college students, primarily the year of study, mathematics background, gender, and the major field of study. The study involved 309 undergraduate students who were enrolled in an introductory statistics course or a college algebra course in the spring 2013 when this study was carried out. According to the findings of this study, the level of anxiety and gender between the students in statistics introductory course and those in the algebra course exhibited demographic differences, primarily on the impact of statistics anxiety and mathematics anxiety on male and female students.

Statistics anxiety did not show statistically significant differences between females and males, t (196) = -0.92, p = 0.36 (Malik, 2014). Similar results on the level of statistics anxiety on gender were obtained by Bui and Alfaro (2011) who used the Test of Science Related Attitudes (TOSRA) and Statistical Anxiety Rating Scale (STARS) to investigate the relationship between statistics anxiety and gender among college students. In this study which comprised of 104 undergraduates, both TOSRA and STARS did not show statistically significant differences, p > .05), between female and males. In contrast, mathematics anxiety was found to have a statistically significant difference between females and males, t (109) = - 2.09, p = 0.04. Second, Malik (2014) found significant differences between the levels of statistics anxiety and mathematics anxiety on the basis of the major field of study. In this context, the researcher investigated anxiety in STEM and non-STEM majors. Results of this

4

study showed that statistics anxiety has a statistically significant difference between STEM and non-STEM majors $F(2, 195) = 12.14$, $p < 0.05$. In contrast, mathematics anxiety did not show statistically significant difference between STEM and non-STEM majors $F(2, 108) = 1.71$, $p = 0.19$. As such, these constructs differed on the two parameters; gender and the major field of study.

On the other hand, there were similarities in the study results on college year and mathematics background. College year did not show statistically significant difference in statistics anxiety between continuing students and freshmen, $t(196) = -1.35$, $p = 0.18$. Similarly, mathematics anxiety did not show statistically significant difference, based on college year, between continuing students and freshmen, $t(109) = -0.30$, $p = 0.76$ (Malik, 2014). Finally, anxiety and mathematics background in both groups showed statistically significant results in which the statistics group had $F(1, 196) = 22.85$, $p < .0001$, whereas the algebra group had $F(1, 109) = 18.15$, $p < .0001$. This implies that mathematics background serves as a significant predictor of both statistics anxiety and mathematics anxiety.

Based on the four parameters of statistics anxiety and mathematics anxiety, the differences of these constructs are conspicuous; thus, clearing the mainstream misconception. Of great importance are the results on anxiety and gender, as well as the field of study which showed significant differences between statistics anxiety and mathematics anxiety (Malik, 2014).

Antecedents of Statistics Anxiety

Over the past few decades, research on statistics anxiety has focused on the underlying causes of the construct (Baloglu, 2004; Zeidner, 1991; Onwuegbuzie, Daros & Ryan, (1997). Baloglu (2004) carried out a comprehensive review of literature that is related to the antecedents of statistics anxiety and noted that it is a multidimensional construct citing Onwuegbuzie, Daros and Ryan's (1997) study that identified instrument anxiety, failure

5

anxiety, interpersonal anxiety, and content anxiety as the main components of statistics anxiety. He identified the main antecedents of this construct as discussed by an array of researchers as environmental, dispositional and situational antecedents. He also found out that some studies regarded statistics anxiety as a bidimensional construct, meaning that it comprises of two dimensions: content anxiety and statistics test anxiety (Zeidner, 1991). However, this aspect was attributable to the fact that these studies did not use statistics anxiety instruments. Instead, they used versions of mathematics anxiety (Baloglu, 2004).

At present, research on the antecedents of statistics anxiety has shifted focus from the predisposing factors to the mechanism involved in the development of statistics anxiety (Macher, Paechter, Papousek & Ruggeri, 2012; Macher et al., 2013). This approach aims at creating advanced understanding on the process of statistics anxiety in order to develop appropriate interventions that will reduce the construct among college students. Recently, Malik (2015) provided an insight into the process of statistics anxiety in which she investigated the underlying factors and situations leading to negative experiences in statistics among college students. In her phenomenological study which involved 6 undergraduate students who were enrolled in an introductory statistics course (STAT 150: Introduction to Statistical Analysis), Malik (2015) was able to investigate the process that leads to negative experiences in statistics. As a methodological approach, the participants were from different fields of study including nursing and psychology, and they were aged 18 years and above. Additionally, this study used students' statistics anxiety scale (SSAS) to carry out a purposeful sampling of participants with high levels of statistics anxiety. According to the findings of Malik's (2015) study, there are situations that induce statistics anxiety among students. She also noted some factors that potentiate statistics anxiety. Other factors that were involved in the development of negative experiences of statistics included feelings of inadequacy, physiological symptoms and the students' inability to conceptualize statistical symbols and terminologies. Based on the four themes, Malik (2015) developed statistics anxiety model of phenomenology that shows how these themes act in a synergistic manner to cause negative experiences on statistics. This model shows giving up as the ultimate outcome.

The Need for Intervention

In retrospect, it is apparent that statistics anxiety has become one of the main barriers in statistics teaching. This aspect is attributable to an array of adverse consequences which are associated with statistics anxiety. Empirical studies indicate that statistics anxiety leads to low statistics performance, negative attitudes towards sciences, as well as self-perception. It also contributes to academic procrastination, one of the major challenging issues in statistics teaching (Onwuegbuzie, 2004).

In prospective study that was conducted by Macher et al. (2013), statistics anxiety was found to be one of the dispositional factors leading to low academic achievement among college students who are enrolled majors that require statistical analysis as part of training. This study was done in Karl-Franzens-University Graz, Austria, and it involved 284 undergraduate students, whose ages ranged between 18 and 46 years. Overall, results of this study indicated that statistics anxiety was negatively related to interest in statistics, $\beta2 =- .21$, as well as academic achievement based on state anxiety, $\beta = -.08$. As such, it was concluded that statistics anxiety influences academic achievement, negatively through inhibiting the decrease of state anxiety during statistics examinations (Macher et al., 2013). Moreover, Onwuegbuzie and Wilson (2003) acknowledge the negative effects of statistics anxiety based on their comprehensive literature review that investigated the causes, effects and treatment of statistics anxiety. Another adverse effect of statistics anxiety is academic procrastination.

According to Onwuegbuzie's (2004) retrospective study that investigated the levels of academic procrastination of the present sample with the norm group that was used in developing Procrastination Assessment Scale-Students (PASS), highly anxious students were fond of procrastination. This study involved 135 graduate students from different graduate-level disciplines. According to the results of this study, it was concluded that statistics anxiety is directly related to academic procrastination (Onwuegbuzie, 2004).

In another study, Perepiczka, Chandler and Becerra (2011) investigated the relationship between statistics anxiety and self-efficacy in statistics and noted a negative correlation. This study involved 166 graduate students were pursuing doctoral and master's programs. Overall, the results of this study revealed that there was a statistically significant correlation between self-efficacy and statistics anxiety, $F(3, 162) = 60.489$, $p < .001$, among graduate students. This implies that statistics anxiety causes negative attitudes towards statistics.

Finally, statistics anxiety has been found to increase intolerance of uncertainty and worry among college students. Williams (2013) investigated the relationship between intolerance of uncertainty, worry and statistics anxiety in a study that involved 97 graduate students from different fields of study including nutritional science, family science, counseling, psychology, and hospitality administration. Based on the results of this study, Williams (2013) concluded that statistics anxiety has a direct relationship with worry among graduate students who are enrolled in statistics-related programs. Therefore, evidence of the negative consequences of statistics anxiety among college students justifies the need for appropriate intervention.

Interventions for Reducing Statistics Anxiety in College Students

Statistics anxiety has been considered as one of the main barriers in achieving success in statistics teaching. As such, ways of reducing statistics anxiety are currently sought in order to enhance statistics teaching through improving students' self-efficacy to learn statistics. This perspective in statistics teaching is based on the rationale that the development of effective statistics anxiety reduction interventions holds the promise for promoting academic achievement, as well as enrollment in statistics related programs in institutions of higher education. To date, an array of intervention strategies that can reduce statistics anxiety among college students have been investigated based on the research findings on the nature of statistics anxiety (Bartsch, Case & Meerman, 2012; Acee & Weinstein, 2010; Ford, Ford, Boxer & Armstrong, 2012; Chiou, Wang & Lee, 2014; Williams, 2010). These involves both cognitive and non-cognitive intervention strategies though majority focus on cognitive perspectives of the construct (Baloglu, 2004).

Use of Live Vicarious Experience Presentation

The use of live vicarious presentation has emerged as one of the most effective ways of reducing statistics anxiety among college students, especially those who are enrolled in research method and statistics courses.

Bartsch, Case and Meerman (2012) investigated the effect of vicarious presentation on increasing students' statistics self-efficacy. This study involved 39 graduate students who were undertaking statistics or research methods courses, and the variables were measured through the use of Self-Efficacy Scale and ANOVA factorials. Overall, the study comprised of two groups; the peer model presentation group and the writing group which did not have live vicarious presentation experience. In principle, researchers in this study carried out pre- and post-interventions to analyze statistics self-efficacy levels between the two groups. A comprehensive analysis of the study results revealed that the experimental (the peer model presentation) has a statistically significant increase in statistics self-efficacy. The pre-intervention self-efficacy was M=6.66 compared to the post intervention level of M=7.07, corresponding to t (19) $=-2.01$, $p =.06$, $d = 0.45$. In contrast, the control group showed a decrease in statistics self-efficacy in pre- and post-intervention results which decreased from

M=6.96 to M=6.48, corresponding to "t (18) = 2.32, p = .03, d = 0.53" (Bartsch, Case & Meerman, 2012, p. 134).

These findings indicate that live vicarious presentations can reduce statistics anxiety because it is indirectly related to statistics self-efficacy. In this context, improving self-efficacy through this approach reduces the adverse effects of the construct.

Value-Reappraisal

Value reappraisal is the second intervention strategy which is considered reliable in reducing statistics anxiety among college students. Evidence for the potential of value reappraisal in reducing statistics anxiety is provided by Acee and Weinstein's (2010) random study that investigated the effects of this strategy on statistics self-efficacy and choice behavior among statistics students. This study comprised of 82 undergraduate students who were taking an introductory statistics course during the fall and spring semesters. In addition, this intervention was provided by two instructors, instructor A and instructor B. Overall, the results of this study revealed that value reappraisal had positive effects on students' choice behavior, endogenous instrumentality, as well as task value. The analysis of the study's data generated high Cronbach's alpha coefficients of the pretest self-report; endogenous instrumentality (.88), task value (.90) and self-efficacy in statistics (.90). In addition, there was a positive correlation between self-efficacy and endogenous instrumentality (r=.26, p<.05) and task value (r=.38, p<.01). Of great interest in this study were the outcomes of Instructor B's students in which the experimental group showed higher post-intervention exam scores in comparison with the control group, "M = 0.62, SE = 0.30, CI = .02 to 1.23, p < .05" (Acee & Weinstein, 2010, p. 504). This indicates that value reappraisal can be an effective strategy for reducing statistics anxiety.

Use of Humor

Humor is known to have significant influence on emotional reactions, as well as cognitive processes (Ford, Ford, Boxer & Armstrong (2012). As such, the incorporation of humor in statistics teaching is becoming of special interest due to its capability of reducing statistics anxiety as it has been proven to do so in mathematics anxiety. Interestingly, humor has been found to reduce state anxiety, an aspect which is caused by both statistics anxiety and mathematics anxiety.

In a prospective study that was carried out by Ford, Ford, Boxer and Armstrong (2012) showed that humor inhibits state anxiety. Participants in this study were 84 in which males were 33, whereas females were 51, all were adult learners enrolled in sociology and psychology courses. The methodological approach involved the exposure of the study participants to 3 conditions of humor manipulation, including funny cartoons, non-humorous poems, and the absence of both in the control group. Overall, humor manipulation was found to have statistically significant effect on state anxiety, F (2, 77) = 6.10, $p < .01$. Participants exposed to the cartoon condition experienced less state anxiety during the test, ($M = 2.77$, $SD = 1.16$) than those in the control group, ($M = 3.93$, $SD = 1.05$). Finally, the regression of state anxiety responses based on humor manipulation was significant, $\beta = .35$, $t = 2.90$, $p < .01$, leading increased academic performance. Conclusively, it is apparent that humor can reduce statistics anxiety due to its positive effect on state anxiety, one of the main aspects of statistics anxiety and mathematics anxiety.

Use of One-Minute Paper Strategy

One-minute paper strategy has been found to be an effective intervention for reducing statistics anxiety among college students enrolled in majors (Chiou, Wang & Lee, 2014). Ideally, one-minute paper strategy involves engaging students in a few minutes' session at the end of each class to answer two questions: "What is the most important concept you learned in class today?" and "What questions remain unanswered?" (Chiou, Wang & Lee, 2014, p. 299). Thereafter, the instructor reads the answers to gauge the students' understanding. Initially, the use of a brief textbook exercise was considered as the most effective strategy, but the one-minute strategy has been found to be more effective in reducing statistics anxiety than the textbook exercise.

Evidence for the effectiveness of the one-minute strategy was provided by a quasi-experimental study that was conducted by Chiou, Wang and Lee (2014) to investigate the effects of the strategy on statistics anxiety and statistics achievement. This study involved 77 undergraduate students who were in the same college year (sophomore) and had similar mathematics background. Participants were also from accounting majors. In approach, the study comprised of the intervention group (30 women, 8 men) and the control group (30 women, 9 men) whose average age was 19.5 years and 19.4 years, respectively. According to the results of this study, the one-minute paper strategy had positive outcomes on statistics achievement and statistics anxiety. In comparison, the experimental group recorded a significant reduction of statistics anxiety than the control group in which their mean differences in posttest and pretest scores were -70.94 and -1.37, respectively. Similarly, the one-minute paper strategy was found to increase statistics achievement over time. Therefore, this strategy was proven to reduce statistics anxiety, as well as enhancing statistics achievement among college students.

Use of Instructor Immediacy

In retrospect, instructor immediacy has received immense focus from researchers in statistics teaching due to its influence on statistics anxiety. Immediacy is a set of communicative behaviors which can influence an individual's perception of psychological and physical closeness (Gorham, 1988). Williams (2010) investigated the influence of instructor immediacy and reported the existence of a positive impact of instructor immediacy on the principal factors of statistics anxiety. She adopted the pretest-posttest-control group methodological design to investigate the construct. Additionally, the researcher used STARS and the Instructor Immediacy scale to measure statistics anxiety and immediacy, respectively. This study involved 76 graduate students, (55 females, 21 males), who were enrolled in an introductory statistics course. According to the results of this study, it was noted that the control group had lower levels of instructor immediacy (M=3.75) than the treatment group (M=4.26), t (74) = 4.48, $p <$ .001. Overall, it was concluded that instructor immediacy is a powerful tool that can reduce statistics anxiety.

Religious Motivation

The effect of religious motivation is explained by the Hope Theory which states the various strategies which are used by an individual to achieve specific life goals. Based on this theory, religious motivation has become one of the main strategies for reducing statistics anxiety among college students. Evidence for effectiveness of religious motivation in reducing statistics anxiety has been investigated in an array of studies. One of these studies is Mvududu and Larocque's (2008) study that examined the relationship between faith, hope and statistics anxiety. Researchers in this study sampled 70 undergraduate students from a secular university (23 students) and a Christian university (47 students) from health science and education majors, who were enrolled in statistics introductory course. Overall, the results of this study indicated that hope is significantly related to religious motivation. In turn, religious motivation was found to have a significant correlation with statistics anxiety. Students from the Christian (Northwest) university had more intrinsic religious motivation, positive attitude, hope, and less statistics anxiety compared to those from the secular (Southeast) university. As such, it was concluded that high intrinsic motivation reduces anxiety levels. Despite, these compelling findings, this study could not be generalized to other populations, and this was one of its limitations. Therefore, future research should focus on promoting the generalizability of these findings through replicating it with other populations, especially non-Christian students attending Christian universities, as well as Christian students in secular universities.

Use of Multifaceted Teaching Framework

Multifaceted teaching framework has been found to be one of the strategies that can reduce statistics anxiety. The effectiveness of this strategy was recently investigated by McGrath et al. (2015) who sought to know how the strategy influenced statistics efficacy among graduate students enrolled in graduate-level statistics course. The researchers recruited 28 graduate students from a Canadian university and employed STARS and the Current Statistics Self-efficacy (CSSE) to measure statistics anxiety and self-efficacy, respectively. As hypothesized, the results of this study revealed that a multifaceted teaching framework increased students' self-efficacy and reduced statistics anxiety. Therefore, these researchers recommended the use of a multifaceted teaching framework for reducing statistics anxiety among graduate students. These results were consistent with the findings of Pan and Tang (2004) who reported a significant relationship between application-oriented methods and statistics anxiety.

Pan and Tang (2004) carried out a prospective study comprising of 21 graduate students who were enrolled in an introductory statistics course. The results of this study showed a significantly correlation between application-oriented teaching strategies and statistics anxiety. The mean scores of the construct in pretest (3.25) and posttest (2.82) showed an empirical reduction of statistics anxiety. These findings provided the initial evidence of the effectiveness of innovative teaching strategies in reducing statistics anxiety.

In-Class Collaborative Problem Solving

In-class collaborative problem-solving may receive increased attention from researchers investigating ways of reducing statistics anxiety among college students. This is attributable to a case study findings reported by Kinkead, Miller and Hammett (2016) who investigated adult perceptions of the intervention. Based on the results of this study, it was found out that majority of the participants considered in-class collaborative problem-solving as a helpful strategy for mitigating statistics anxiety. Of the 14 participants, 10 (71%) considered this approach as helpful compared to 4 (29%) who perceived it marginal or problematic. It is imperative that the perceptions of those who did not consider in-class collaborative problem-solving as helpful in reducing statistics anxiety were influenced by other factors such as partner compatibility. These findings set the foundation for further research on the effect of in-class collaborative problem-solving in reducing statistics anxiety.

It is apparent that the adult perceptions reported from the case study advances the recommendations of the 2007 American Sociological Association teaching workshop that highlighted on several strategies that can reduce students' anxieties through collaborative classroom environment. Macheski, Buhrmann, Lowney and Bush (2008) elucidate the resolutions of this conference which was dubbed "Innovative Teaching Practices for Difficult Subjects." The main theme of this conference was on 'building a community of learners' in statistics, research methods and theory courses by all faculties. As discussed in the conference, the process of building a collaborative learning environment requires the faculties to create and maintain: "1) an active role for students; 2) a common language of discourse; and 3) a supportive emotional environment" (p. 45). As such, it is apparent that these aspects will enhance students' engagement and reduce statistics anxiety.

Use of Technology (Web-based Instruction)

Web-based instruction may gain popularity as an effective tool for reducing anxiety among statistics students following the findings of Gundy, Liu, Morton and Kline (2006). However, most researchers have investigated the effects of this aspect on mathematics anxiety, but not statistics anxiety. Nevertheless, the positive effects of web-based instruction recorded in students experiencing mathematics anxiety have immense significance on reducing statistics anxiety. In this context, the outcomes of Gundy, Liu, Morton and Kline's (2006) quasi-experiment that investigated the relationship between students' self-esteem, sense of mastery, mathematics anxiety and web-based instruction provide revelations of its usefulness for reducing statistics anxiety too. Additionally, the fact that the participants in this study were undergraduate statistics students potentiates its relevance of in statistics teaching. The study involved 175 students as participants, and it comprised of three study conditions: condition A, B and C in which the intervention was tested. Overall, the results of this study showed an increase in the students' sense of mastery, self-esteem and reduced levels mathematics anxiety. This suggests that web-based instruction can be helpful in reducing statistics anxiety within this students group.

Combined Instructional Strategies

Other instructional methods which have been found to reduce statistics anxiety in college students include SPSS assignments, readings, in-class demonstration, and student's presentation as reported by Quinn (2006). This study involved 13 participants who were enrolled in a statistics course. Overall, these instructional methods were found to reduce statistics anxiety. The means score differences between the pretests and posttests showed a reduction by 13.75 points.

Summary of Literature on Statistics Anxiety Interventions

Conclusively, this review of literature shows the existence of vast interventions that can reduce statistics anxiety in college students. Some of these interventions include live vicarious presentation (Bartsch, Case & Meerman, 2012), value reappraisal (Acee & Weinstein, 2010), humor (Ford, Ford, Boxer & Armstrong, 2012), one-minute paper strategy (Chiou, Wang & Lee, 2014), instructor immediacy (Williams, 2010), and multifaceted teaching framework (McGrath et al., 2015; Pan & Tang, 2004). Other teaching strategies for reducing statistics anxiety are religious motivation (Mvududu & Larocque, 2008), web-based instruction (Gundy, Liu, Morton & Kline, 2006) and in-class collaborative problem-solving (Macheski, Buhrmann, Lowney & Bush, 2008; Kinkead, Miller & Hammett, 2016).

References

Acee, T. W., & Weinstein, C. E. (2010). Effects of a Value-Reappraisal Intervention on Statistics Students' Motivation and Performance. *The Journal of Experimental Education, 78*, 487–512. doi: 10.1080/00220970903352753

Baloglu, M. (2004). Statistics anxiety and mathematics anxiety: Some interesting differences. *Educational Research Quarterly, 27*(3), 38-48.

Bartsch, R. A., Case, K. A., & Meerman, H. (2012). Increasing academic self-efficacy in statistics with a live vicarious experience presentation. *Teaching of Psychology 39*(2), 133-136. doi: 10.1177/0098628312437699

Bui, N. H., & Alfaro, M. A. (2011). Statistics anxiety and science attitudes: Age, gender, and ethnicity factors. *College Student Journal, 45*(3), 573–585.

Chiou, C., Wang, Y., & Lee, L. (2014). Reducing statistics anxiety and enhancing statistics learning achievement: effectiveness of a one-minute strategy. *Psychological Reports: Sociocultural Issues in Psychology, 115*(1), 297-310. doi: 10.2466/11.04.PR0.115c12z3

Cruise, J. R., Cash, R. W., & Bolton, L. D. (1985). Development and validation of an instrument to measure statistical anxiety. In ASA Proceedings (Ed.), *Statistical education section* (pp. 92-98). Washington, Washington, DC: American Statistical Association.

Dykeman, B. F. (2011). Statistics anxiety: antecedents and instructional interventions. *Education, 132*(2), 441-446.

Ford, T. E., Ford, B. L., Boxer, C. F., & Armstrong, J. (2012). Effect of humor on state anxiety and math performance. *Humor, 25*(1), 59-74. doi: 10.1515/humor-2012-0004

Gorham, J. (1988). The relationship between verbal teacher immediacy behaviors and student learning. *Communication Education, 37*, 40-53.

Gundy, K., Liu, H. Q., Morton, B. A., & Kline, J. (2006). Effects of Web-Based Instruction on Math Anxiety, the Sense of Mastery, and Global Self-Esteem: A Quasi-Experimental Study of Undergraduate Statistics Students. *Teaching Sociology, 34*, 370-388.

Hak, A. (2014). *Combating math anxiety: taking a look into teacher perceptions regarding the use of technology in elementary math classrooms* (Master's Thesis. University of Toronto, Toronto, Canada). Retrieved from https://tspace.library.utoronto.ca/bitstream/1807/67026/1/Hak_%20Ameena_2014June_MT_MTRP.pdf

Kinkead, K. J., Miller, H., & Hammett, R. (2016). Adult perceptions of in-class collaborative problem solving as mitigation for statistics anxiety. *The Journal of Continuing Higher Education, 64*(2), 101-111. doi: 10.1080/07377363.2016.1178057

Macher, D., Paechter, M., Papousek, I., & Ruggeri, K. (2012). Statistics anxiety, trait anxiety, learning behavior, and academic performance. *European Journal of Psychology of Education, 27*(4), 483–498. doi:10.1007/s10212-011-0090-5

Macher, D., Paechter, M., Papousek, I., Ruggeri, K., Freudenthaler, H. H., & Arendasy, M. (2013). Statistics anxiety, state anxiety during an examination, and academic achievement. *British Journal of Educational Psychology, 83*, 535–549.

Macheski, G. E., Buhrmann, J., Lowney, K. S., & Bush, M. E. (2008). Overcoming student disengagement and anxiety in theory, methods, and statistics courses by building a community of learners. *Teaching Sociology, 36*, 42-48.

Malik, S. (2014). Undergraduates' Statistics Anxiety and Mathematics Anxiety: Are They Similar or Different Constructs? *JSM*. Retrieved from https://www.amstat.org/sections/srms/proceedings/y2014/files/311309_87289.pdf

Malik, S. (2015).Undergraduates' statistics anxiety: A phenomenological study. *The Qualitative Report, 20*(2), 120-133.

McGrath, A. L., Ferns, A., Greiner, L., Wanamaker, K., & Brown, S. (2015). Reducing Anxiety and Increasing Self-efficacy within an Advanced Graduate Psychology Statistics Course. *The Canadian Journal for the Scholarship of Teaching and Learning, 6*(1), 1-17. doi: http://dx.doi.org/10.5206/cjsotl-rcacea.2015.1.5

Mvududu, N., & Larocque, M. (2008). Hope, faith, and statistics: an examination of the relationship. *Christian Higher Education, 7,* 171–184. doi: 10.1080/15363750801891069

Onwuegbuzie, A. J. (2004). Academic procrastination and statistics anxiety. *Assessment & Evaluation in Higher Education, 29*(1), 1-19.

Onwuegbuzie, A. J., & Wilson, V. A. (2003). Statistics Anxiety: nature, etiology, antecedents, effects, and treatments—a comprehensive review of the literature. *Teaching in Higher Education, 8*(2), 195–209.

Onwuegbuzie, A. J., Daros, D., & Ryan, J. (1997). The components of statistics anxiety: a phenomenological study. *Focus on Learning Problems in Mathematics, 19*(4), 11–35.

Pan, W., & Tang, M. (2004). Examining the effectiveness of innovative instructional methods on reducing statistics anxiety for graduate students in the social sciences. *Journal of Instructional Psychology, 31*(2), 149-159.

Perepiczka, M., Chandler, N., & Becerra, M. (2011). Relationship between graduate students' statistics self-efficacy, statistics anxiety, attitude toward statistics, and social support. *The Professional Counselor, 1*(2), 99-108. doi:10.15241/mpa.1.2.99

Quinn, A. (2006). Reducing social work students' statistics anxiety. *Academic Exchange Quarterly, 10*(2), 167-171. Retrieved from http://und.edu/instruct/aquinn/academic_exchange_quinn.pdf

Williams, A. S. (2010). Statistics anxiety and instructor immediacy. *Journal of Statistics Education, 18*(2), 1-18.

Williams, A. S. (2013). Worry, intolerance of uncertainty, and statistics anxiety. *Statistics Education Research Journal, 12*(1), 48-59.

Zeidner, M. (1991). Statistics and mathematics anxiety in social science students—some interesting parallels. *British Journal of Educational Psychology, 61*, 319–328.

Zerbolio, D. J. (1999). A bag of tricks for teaching about sampling distributions. In M. E. Ware & C. L. Brewer (Eds.), *Handbook for teaching statistics and research methods* (2nd ed.). New Jersey, NJ: Lawrence Erlbaum Associates, Publishers.

YOUR KNOWLEDGE HAS VALUE

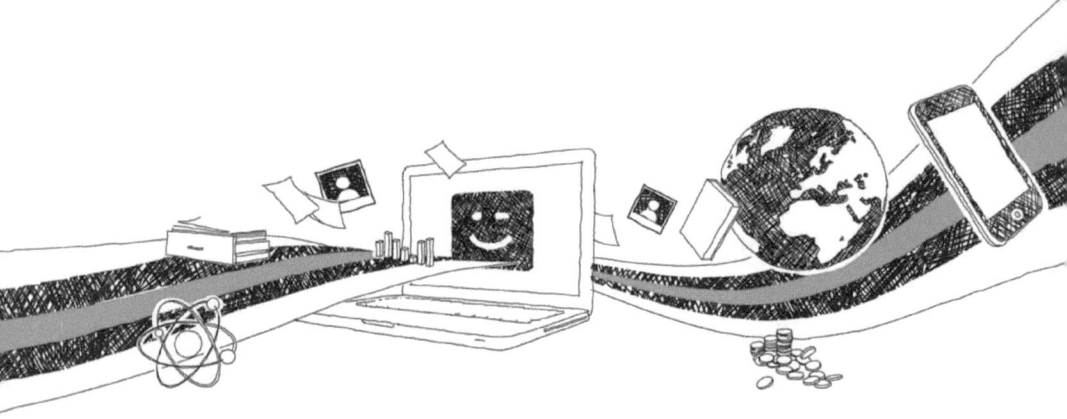

- We will publish your bachelor's and master's thesis, essays and papers

- Your own eBook and book - sold worldwide in all relevant shops

- Earn money with each sale

Upload your text at www.GRIN.com and publish for free

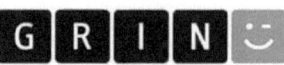